THE COMPLETE ARTHRITIS DIET COOKBOOK FOR ADULT

From Joint-Friendly Delights to Nutritional Triumphs: A Culinary Odyssey for Arthritis Well-Being

Jose Williams

Disclaimer Statement

Please keep in mind that the contents of this booklet are meant for educational and recreational purposes. Every effort has been made to offer accurate, up-to-date, reliable, and thorough information. There are, however, no stated or implied assurances of any kind. Readers understand that the author is providing competent counsel. The content in this book originates from several sources. Please seek the opinion of a competent professional before using any of the tactics outlined in this book. By reading this book, the reader agrees that the author will not be held accountable for any direct or indirect damages resulting from the use of the information contained therein, including, but not limited to, errors, omissions, or inaccuracies.

Table of Contents

INTRODUCTION

Dear Reader, if you've ever found yourself caught in the labyrinth of arthritis, navigating a terrain where every step is a reminder of your body's unique challenges, welcome. You're not alone. In fact, you're in the company of someone who knows those creaks and groans all too well, and I'm here to be your culinary comrade on this extraordinary journey.

Arthritis, with its unpredictable twists and turns, can feel like a capricious dance partner, leading you into steps you never anticipated. I get it. Those moments of frustration, the silent negotiations with your body, and the occasional eye roll when yet another joint decides to add its voice to the chorus – they're not lost on me. If arthritis were a board game, it would be the one with an ever-changing maze, and the finish line seems to move just when you think you've got the hang of it.

So, why a cookbook? Because sometimes, the most comforting moments are found in the rhythm of a whisk, the sizzle of a pan, and the aroma of a well-seasoned dish. This is not just a collection of recipes; it's a culinary companion crafted with empathy, a sprinkling of humor, and an understanding that goes beyond the ingredients.

Before we embark on our culinary adventure, let's have an honest conversation about arthritis and nutrition. Think of it as sitting down with a friend who knows the intricacies of the journey you're on. Arthritis isn't a one-size-fits-all scenario; it's a nuanced tapestry woven with the threads of your unique experiences.

It's like trying to solve a puzzle, and the pieces are scattered across the table. Some days, the picture becomes clearer, and on others, it feels like the pieces are mocking you from their scattered positions. But here's the thing – we're in this puzzle-solving business together.

Understanding the science behind arthritis and its connection to what we put on our plates is not about turning you into a nutrition expert. It's about arming you with the knowledge to make informed choices. So, brace yourself – not just for the pun, but for a journey through the intricacies of arthritis, where science meets the art of cooking.

Now, let's talk about your kitchen – the battleground for your culinary adventures. Have you ever felt like your pantry is a magical realm where ingredients appear and disappear at will? If finding that elusive spice feels like a quest of mythical proportions, you're not alone.

A pantry makeover is not just about organizing shelves; it's a declaration of war against chaos. It's reclaiming your kitchen, turning it into a space where every ingredient has a purpose and a story. Imagine it as a quest for the Holy Grail – only, in this case, the grail is a well-organized spice rack, and the victory cry is more of a satisfied sigh.

Mornings can be a bit of a battlefield, can't they? The alarm clock is the bugle call, and the kitchen is the war room where you plan your first nutritional assault on the day. Breakfast is the hero in this saga, the meal that sets the tone for the rest of your culinary adventures.

Whether you're a breakfast champion or a reluctant riser, our journey into morning delights is about infusing your day with flavors that inspire. It's not just about nourishing your body; it's about feeding your soul, preparing you for the day's battles armed with a satisfied stomach and a smile.

Lunchtime, the unsung hero of the daily narrative. It's not just about refueling; it's a chance to pause, regroup, and savor the flavors of a well-crafted meal. Picture it as a midday oasis, a moment of respite from the demands of the world.

This chapter is not just about recipes; it's about transforming lunch from a routine to a ritual. It's about finding joy in the simplicity of a well-prepared dish, a moment of calm before you dive back into the whirlwind of life.

Evenings are for winding down, and dinner should be the supporting actor in this nightly drama. Think of it as the backdrop to the closing scenes of your day, providing comfort, nourishment, and perhaps a touch of culinary magic.

Dinner in the world of arthritis isn't just about filling your stomach; it's about creating dishes that provide the extra care your body deserves. It's a culinary embrace, a warm hug at the end of a day that may have thrown a few unexpected curveballs your way.

Snacking often gets a bad rap, doesn't it? But what if I told you that snacking could be a joyful experience, a moment of pleasure without the guilt? It's like finding the sweet spot between indulgence and nourishment, where each bite is a celebration of flavors and well-being.

This chapter is all about mastering the art of snacking, turning mindless munching into a purposeful and delightful experience. Because, let's be honest, life is too short for tasteless snacks.

Ah, desserts – the grand finale of any culinary journey. Life is too short to skip the sweet moments, but it's also too precious to compromise your well-being. In this chapter, we'll embark on a guilt-free journey through the world of indulgent desserts.

Picture it as the cherry on top of a delicious cake, the moment when you savor the sweetness of life without sacrificing your health goals. Desserts, when done right, can be the perfect exclamation point to a well-lived day.

Dear friend, as I share these recipes and stories with you, I want you to know that I'm not just a voice on these pages. I'm a friend who understands the language of arthritis, the nuances of its challenges, and the victories, however small, that come with each day.

Arthritis isn't just a physical battle; it's a journey that tests your resilience, challenges your spirit, and sometimes, makes you question the fairness of it all. But through the tapestry of challenges, there's an opportunity to find joy, to savor the moments of triumph, and to appreciate the simple pleasures that a well-prepared meal can bring.

So, as you dive into these pages, imagine me standing there with you in the kitchen, apron on, ready to share a laugh, a piece of advice, or simply a quiet moment of understanding. We're in this together, navigating the culinary landscape with laughter, compassion, and a pinch of spice.

This cookbook is not just a collection of recipes; it's a culinary confidante, a companion on your journey to better health. Let's make cooking not just a necessity but a joyful celebration of life. Here's to delicious meals, pain-free days, and the beautiful journey we're about to embark on together.

Warmly,

ARTHRITIS-FRIENDLY INGREDIENTS

In the realm of arthritis-friendly cooking, understanding the impact of ingredients on joint health is paramount. As a nutritionist with a keen interest in optimizing well-being through diet, I am excited to guide you through the essential components of an arthritis-friendly pantry. Our journey will explore vital nutrients for joint health, delve into the benefits of omega-3 fatty acids, antioxidants, and various vitamins and minerals. Additionally, we'll discuss practical ingredient substitutions for arthritis-friendly cooking, focusing on healthy fats, low-impact carbohydrates, and lean proteins.

Essential Nutrients for Joint Health

When it comes to promoting joint health, a well-rounded diet is your greatest ally. Essential nutrients play a pivotal role in maintaining the integrity of your joints and mitigating inflammation. Incorporating a variety of these nutrients into your meals can contribute to the overall health of your joints.

Omega-3 Fatty Acids

- Omega-3 fatty acids are like superheroes for your joints. Found in fatty fish like salmon, mackerel, and flaxseeds, these fatty acids possess potent anti-inflammatory properties. They help reduce joint stiffness and pain, making them an indispensable part of an arthritis-friendly diet. Consider incorporating fatty fish into your weekly meals or adding flaxseeds to your morning smoothie for a delightful omega-3 boost.

Antioxidants

- Imagine antioxidants as the shield that guards your joints from oxidative stress. Berries, leafy greens, and colorful vegetables are rich in antioxidants, providing essential protection against inflammation. Including a vibrant array of fruits and vegetables in your daily meals not only enhances the flavor but also nourishes your joints from within.

Vitamins and Minerals

- Certain vitamins and minerals act as crucial players in the joint health game. Vitamin C, abundant in citrus fruits and bell peppers, aids in collagen formation, essential for maintaining joint structure. Vitamin D, often obtained through sunlight or fortified foods, supports calcium absorption, contributing to bone health. Additionally, minerals like calcium and magnesium play pivotal roles in maintaining bone density and muscle function.

Ingredient Substitutions for Arthritis-Friendly Cooking

Making your kitchen arthritis-friendly involves not just what you include but also what you choose to exclude or substitute. Let's explore some smart ingredient swaps that can enhance the nutritional profile of your meals without compromising on flavor.

Healthy Fats

- While fats have long been misunderstood, the truth is, they are essential for overall health, especially for those with arthritis. Opt for heart-healthy fats like olive oil, avocado, and nuts. These fats not only add a delightful richness to your dishes but also bring anti-inflammatory benefits to the table.

Low-Impact Carbohydrates

- Carbohydrates are a fundamental source of energy, but not all carbs are created equal. Choose complex carbohydrates like quinoa, sweet potatoes, and whole grains. These low-impact options provide sustained energy without causing spikes in blood sugar levels, which can be beneficial for managing arthritis symptoms.

Lean Proteins

- Protein is a crucial building block for your body, aiding in muscle repair and overall well-being. Opt for lean protein sources such as poultry, fish, tofu, and legumes. These options provide ample protein without the added burden of excessive saturated fats, supporting your joint health goals.
- In the pursuit of an arthritis-friendly kitchen, these substitutions not only contribute to joint health but also enhance the overall nutritional value of your meals.
- As we continue our culinary exploration, keep in mind that these aren't rigid rules but rather adaptable guidelines. Feel free to experiment and tailor these suggestions to suit your personal preferences and dietary needs.
- In essence, arthritis-friendly cooking is not about sacrifice but about making informed choices that resonate with your body's unique requirements. By embracing these nutrient-rich ingredients and smart substitutions, you're not just crafting delicious meals – you're nurturing your joints from the inside out.
- Remember, the journey to optimal joint health is a marathon, not a sprint. Small, sustainable changes in your dietary choices can

lead to significant improvements over time. So, let's embark on this flavorful expedition together, discovering the joy of arthritis-friendly cooking one nutritious bite at a time.

BREAKFAST RECIPES

Blueberry Almond Chia Pudding Bowl

Prep Time: 10 mins

Total Time: 4 hours (including chilling time)

Servings: 2 bowls

Ingredients:

- 1 cup almond milk
- 1/4 cup chia seeds
- 1/2 teaspoon vanilla extract
- 1 tablespoon maple syrup
- 1/2 cup fresh blueberries
- 1/4 cup sliced almonds
- Fresh mint leaves for garnish

Directions:

1. In a bowl, whisk together almond milk, chia seeds, vanilla extract, and maple syrup.
2. Let the mixture sit for 5 minutes, then whisk again to prevent clumping.
3. Cover the bowl and refrigerate for at least 4 hours or overnight.
4. Before serving, stir the chia pudding to ensure an even consistency.
5. Divide the pudding into two bowls and top with fresh blueberries, sliced almonds, and mint leaves.

Nutritional Information (per serving):

- Calories: 270

- Protein: 6g
- Fat: 15g
- Carbohydrates: 29g
- Fiber: 12g
- Sugars: 10g

Spinach and Feta Omelette

Prep Time: 5 mins

Total Time: 10 mins

Servings: 1 omelette

Ingredients:

- 2 large eggs
- 1/4 cup fresh spinach, chopped
- 2 tablespoons feta cheese, crumbled
- 1 teaspoon olive oil
- Salt and pepper to taste
- Fresh herbs (such as parsley or chives) for garnish

Directions:

1. In a bowl, whisk together the eggs and season with salt and pepper.
2. Heat olive oil in a non-stick pan over medium heat.
3. Add chopped spinach to the pan and cook for 1-2 minutes until wilted.
4. Pour the whisked eggs over the spinach, letting them set slightly.
5. Sprinkle feta cheese over one half of the omelette and fold the other half over the filling.

6. Cook for an additional 2-3 minutes until the eggs are fully cooked.

7. Garnish with fresh herbs and serve.

Nutritional Information (per serving):

- Calories: 320
- Protein: 20g
- Fat: 24g
- Carbohydrates: 4g
- Fiber: 1g
- Sugars: 2g

Quinoa Breakfast Bowl

Prep Time: 10 mins

Total Time: 20 mins

Servings: 2 bowls

Ingredients:

- 1 cup cooked quinoa
- 1/2 cup Greek yogurt
- 1 tablespoon honey
- 1/4 cup sliced strawberries
- 1/4 cup blueberries
- 1 tablespoon chia seeds
- 1 tablespoon chopped nuts (almonds, walnuts, or pistachios)

Directions:

1. In a bowl, combine cooked quinoa and Greek yogurt.

2. Drizzle honey over the mixture and stir to combine.

3. Divide the quinoa mixture into two bowls.

4. Top each bowl with sliced strawberries, blueberries, chia seeds, and chopped nuts.

Nutritional Information (per serving):

- Calories: 280
- Protein: 12g
- Fat: 7g
- Carbohydrates: 45g
- Fiber: 6g
- Sugars: 17g

Avocado and Smoked Salmon Toast

Prep Time: 8 mins

Total Time: 10 mins

Servings: 2 slices

Ingredients:

- 2 slices whole-grain bread
- 1 ripe avocado
- 4 ounces smoked salmon
- 1 tablespoon capers
- Lemon wedges for serving
- Fresh dill for garnish

Directions:

1. Toast the slices of whole-grain bread to your liking.
2. Mash the ripe avocado and spread it evenly over the toasted bread.
3. Arrange smoked salmon on top of the avocado.
4. Sprinkle capers over the salmon.

5. Garnish with fresh dill and serve with lemon wedges on the side.

Nutritional Information (per serving):

- Calories: 320
- Protein: 18g
- Fat: 18g
- Carbohydrates: 25g
- Fiber: 8g
- Sugars: 1g

Berry and Almond Smoothie Bowl

Prep Time: 5 mins

Total Time: 5 mins

Servings: 1 bowl

Ingredients:

- 1 cup frozen mixed berries (blueberries, strawberries, raspberries)
- 1/2 banana
- 1/2 cup almond milk
- 1 tablespoon almond butter
- 1 tablespoon chia seeds
- Fresh berries and sliced almonds for topping

Directions:

1. In a blender, combine frozen berries, banana, almond milk, almond butter, and chia seeds.
2. Blend until smooth and creamy.
3. Pour the smoothie into a bowl.

4. Top with fresh berries and sliced almonds.

Nutritional Information (per serving):

- Calories: 310
- Protein: 8g
- Fat: 16g
- Carbohydrates: 38g
- Fiber: 12g
- Sugars: 18g

Golden Turmeric Oatmeal Bowl

Prep Time: 5 mins

Total Time: 10 mins

Servings: 2 bowls

Ingredients:

- 1 cup old-fashioned oats
- 2 cups almond milk
- 1 teaspoon ground turmeric
- 1/2 teaspoon cinnamon
- 1 tablespoon chia seeds
- 1/4 cup chopped walnuts
- 1 tablespoon honey or maple syrup (optional)
- Fresh berries for topping

Directions:

1. In a saucepan, combine oats, almond milk, turmeric, and cinnamon.

2. Cook over medium heat, stirring occasionally, until the oats are tender.

3. Stir in chia seeds, chopped walnuts, and sweetener if desired.

4. Divide the oatmeal into two bowls and top with fresh berries.

Nutritional Information (per serving):

- Calories: 320

- Protein: 9g

- Fat: 15g

- Carbohydrates: 43g

- Fiber: 9g

- Sugars: 8g

Mango Avocado Breakfast Parfait

Prep Time: 10 mins

Total Time: 10 mins

Servings: 2 parfaits

Ingredients:

- 1 ripe mango, diced

- 1 ripe avocado, diced

- 1 cup Greek yogurt

- 1/2 cup granola (choose a low-sugar option)

- 2 tablespoons honey

- 1/4 cup chopped almonds

- Fresh mint leaves for garnish

Directions:

1. In a glass or bowl, layer diced mango, diced avocado, and Greek yogurt.

2. Sprinkle granola over the yogurt layer.

3. Drizzle honey over the granola.

4. Top with chopped almonds and garnish with fresh mint leaves.

Nutritional Information (per serving):

- Calories: 380
- Protein: 15g
- Fat: 20g
- Carbohydrates: 40g
- Fiber: 7g
- Sugars: 24g

Salmon and Avocado Breakfast Wrap

Prep Time: 10 mins

Total Time: 15 mins

Servings: 2 wraps

Ingredients:

- 2 whole-grain tortillas
- 4 ounces smoked salmon
- 1 ripe avocado, sliced
- 1 tablespoon cream cheese
- 1 tablespoon capers
- Fresh dill for garnish

Directions:

1. Lay out the tortillas and spread cream cheese over each.
2. Arrange smoked salmon slices on one half of each tortilla.
3. Add sliced avocado and sprinkle capers over the salmon.
4. Garnish with fresh dill and fold the tortillas in half to create wraps.

Nutritional Information (per serving):

- Calories: 290

- Protein: 15g

- Fat: 15g

- Carbohydrates: 24g

- Fiber: 6g

- Sugars: 2g

Sweet Potato and Spinach Breakfast Hash

Prep Time: 15 mins

Total Time: 25 mins

Servings: 2 servings

Ingredients:

- 2 medium sweet potatoes, peeled and diced

- 1 cup fresh spinach, chopped

- 1 tablespoon olive oil

- 1/2 teaspoon paprika

- 1/4 teaspoon garlic powder

- Salt and pepper to taste

- 2 eggs (optional, for serving)

Directions:

1. In a skillet, heat olive oil over medium heat.

2. Add diced sweet potatoes and cook until tender.

3. Stir in chopped spinach, paprika, garlic powder, salt, and pepper.

4. If desired, cook eggs sunny-side-up in the same skillet.

5. Divide the sweet potato and spinach hash between two plates and top with optional eggs.

Nutritional Information (per serving, without eggs):

- Calories: 230
- Protein: 4g
- Fat: 7g
- Carbohydrates: 40g
- Fiber: 6g
- Sugars: 9g

Protein-Packed Greek Yogurt Bowl

Prep Time: 5 mins

Total Time: 5 mins

Servings: 1 bowl

Ingredients:

- 1 cup Greek yogurt
- 1/2 cup mixed berries (blueberries, strawberries)
- 1 tablespoon almond butter
- 1 tablespoon chia seeds
- 1 tablespoon honey
- 1/4 cup granola

Directions:

1. In a bowl, layer Greek yogurt.
2. Top with mixed berries, almond butter, chia seeds, and honey.
3. Sprinkle granola over the top for added crunch.

Nutritional Information (per serving):

- Calories: 380
- Protein: 20g
- Fat: 15g

- Carbohydrates: 45g

- Fiber: 7g

- Sugars: 30g

Quinoa Breakfast Bowl

Prep Time: 5 mins

Total Time: 20 mins

Servings: 2 bowls

Ingredients:

- 1/2 cup quinoa, rinsed

- 1 cup almond milk

- 1/2 teaspoon cinnamon

- 1 tablespoon chia seeds

- 1/4 cup sliced almonds

- 1 cup mixed berries (blueberries, strawberries)

- 1 tablespoon honey or maple syrup

Directions:

1. In a saucepan, combine quinoa, almond milk, and cinnamon.

2. Bring to a boil, then reduce heat, cover, and simmer for 15 minutes or until quinoa is cooked.

3. Stir in chia seeds and let it sit for 5 minutes.

4. Fluff the quinoa with a fork and divide into two bowls.

5. Top with sliced almonds, mixed berries, and drizzle with honey or maple syrup.

Nutritional Information (per serving):

- Calories: 320

- Protein: 9g

- Fat: 11g

- Carbohydrates: 48g

- Fiber: 8g

- Sugars: 18g

Sweet Potato and Spinach Omelette

Prep Time: 10 mins

Total Time: 15 mins

Servings: 1 omelette

Ingredients:

- 2 eggs

- 1/4 cup cooked sweet potato, diced

- 1/2 cup fresh spinach, chopped

- 1 tablespoon feta cheese, crumbled

- 1 teaspoon olive oil

- Salt and pepper to taste

Directions:

1. In a bowl, beat the eggs and season with salt and pepper.

2. Heat olive oil in a non-stick pan over medium heat.

3. Add sweet potato and spinach to the pan, cooking until spinach wilts.

4. Pour the beaten eggs over the vegetables.

5. Sprinkle feta cheese over one half of the omelette and fold the other half over the filling.

6. Cook for 2-3 minutes until the eggs are fully cooked.

Nutritional Information (per serving):

- Calories: 290

- Protein: 18g
- Fat: 20g
- Carbohydrates: 12g
- Fiber: 2g
- Sugars: 2g

Chia Seed Pudding with Berries

Prep Time: 5 mins (plus chilling time)

Total Time: 4 hours

Servings: 2 bowls

Ingredients:

- 1/4 cup chia seeds
- 1 cup almond milk
- 1/2 teaspoon vanilla extract
- 1 tablespoon maple syrup
- 1 cup mixed berries (strawberries, raspberries, blueberries)
- 2 tablespoons sliced almonds

Directions:

1. In a bowl, whisk together chia seeds, almond milk, vanilla extract, and maple syrup.
2. Let the mixture sit for 5 minutes, then whisk again to prevent clumping.
3. Cover the bowl and refrigerate for at least 4 hours or overnight.
4. Before serving, stir the chia pudding to ensure an even consistency.
5. Divide the pudding into two bowls and top with mixed berries and sliced almonds.

Nutritional Information (per serving):

- Calories: 220
- Protein: 7g
- Fat: 11g
- Carbohydrates: 28g
- Fiber: 11g
- Sugars: 12g

Avocado and Berry Smoothie

Prep Time: 5 mins

Total Time: 5 mins

Servings: 2 glasses

Ingredients:

- 1 ripe avocado
- 1 cup mixed berries (blueberries, raspberries, strawberries)
- 1 cup coconut water or almond milk
- 1 tablespoon chia seeds
- 1 tablespoon honey
- 1/2 cup ice cubes

Directions:

1. In a blender, combine the ripe avocado, mixed berries, coconut water or almond milk, chia seeds, honey, and ice cubes.
2. Blend until smooth and creamy.
3. Pour the smoothie into two glasses and serve immediately.

Nutritional Information (per serving):

- Calories: 260
- Protein: 4g

- Fat: 14g

- Carbohydrates: 33g

- Fiber: 9g

- Sugars: 20g

Smoked Salmon and Cucumber Bagel

Prep Time: 10 mins

Total Time: 15 mins

Servings: 1 bagel

Ingredients:

- 1 whole-grain bagel

- 2 ounces smoked salmon

- 1/4 cup Greek yogurt

- 1/4 cucumber, thinly sliced

- Fresh dill for garnish

- Lemon wedges for serving

Directions:

1. Toast the whole-grain bagel to your liking.

2. Spread Greek yogurt on each half of the bagel.

3. Arrange smoked salmon over the yogurt.

4. Top with thinly sliced cucumber and garnish with fresh dill.

5. Serve with lemon wedges on the side.

Nutritional Information (per serving):

- Calories: 340

- Protein: 25g

- Fat: 12g

- Carbohydrates: 35g

- Fiber: 5g

- Sugars: 4g

Arthritis-Busting Berry Smoothie Bowl

Prep Time: 10 mins

Total Time: 10 mins

Servings: 1 bowl

Ingredients:

- 1 cup mixed frozen berries (blueberries, strawberries, raspberries)
- 1/2 banana
- 1/2 cup almond milk
- 1 tablespoon chia seeds
- 1 tablespoon almond butter
- 1 teaspoon honey
- 1/4 cup granola
- Fresh mint leaves for garnish

Directions:

1. In a blender, combine mixed berries, banana, almond milk, chia seeds, and almond butter.
2. Blend until smooth and creamy.
3. Pour the smoothie into a bowl.
4. Drizzle honey over the top and sprinkle with granola.
5. Garnish with fresh mint leaves.

Nutritional Information (per serving):

- Calories: 340
- Protein: 9g

- Fat: 14g
- Carbohydrates: 48g
- Fiber: 10g
- Sugars: 22g

Turmeric-Infused Scrambled Eggs with Spinach

Prep Time: 5 mins

Total Time: 10 mins

Servings: 1 serving

Ingredients:

- 2 large eggs
- 1/2 teaspoon ground turmeric
- 1 cup fresh spinach, chopped
- 1 teaspoon olive oil
- Salt and pepper to taste
- Fresh herbs for garnish (parsley or cilantro)

Directions:

1. In a bowl, whisk together eggs and ground turmeric. Season with salt and pepper.
2. Heat olive oil in a pan over medium heat.
3. Add chopped spinach to the pan and sauté until wilted.
4. Pour the whisked eggs over the spinach and scramble until fully cooked.
5. Garnish with fresh herbs before serving.

Nutritional Information (per serving):

- Calories: 280
- Protein: 17g

- Fat: 20g

- Carbohydrates: 4g

- Fiber: 2g

- Sugars: 1g

Chia Seed and Coconut Yogurt Parfait

Prep Time: 5 mins (plus chilling time)

Total Time: 4 hours

Servings: 2 parfaits

Ingredients:

- 1/2 cup chia seeds

- 1 1/2 cups coconut yogurt

- 1 cup mixed tropical fruits (pineapple, mango, kiwi)

- 2 tablespoons shredded coconut

- 1 tablespoon agave syrup

Directions:

1. In a bowl, mix chia seeds and coconut yogurt. Refrigerate for at least 4 hours or overnight.

2. Layer chia pudding, mixed tropical fruits, and shredded coconut in glasses.

3. Drizzle agave syrup over each layer.

4. Repeat the layers until the glasses are filled.

Nutritional Information (per serving):

- Calories: 320

- Protein: 9g

- Fat: 14g

- Carbohydrates: 42g

- Fiber: 14g

- Sugars: 20g

Salmon and Avocado Breakfast Salad

Prep Time: 15 mins

Total Time: 15 mins

Servings: 1 salad

Ingredients:

- 4 ounces smoked salmon

- 1/2 avocado, sliced

- 1 cup mixed greens (kale, spinach, arugula)

- 1 tablespoon olive oil

- 1 tablespoon lemon juice

- Salt and pepper to taste

- 1 boiled egg, sliced

Directions:

1. Arrange mixed greens on a plate.

2. Top with smoked salmon and sliced avocado.

3. Drizzle olive oil and lemon juice over the salad.

4. Season with salt and pepper.

5. Garnish with sliced boiled egg.

Nutritional Information (per serving):

- Calories: 350

- Protein: 22g

- Fat: 25g

- Carbohydrates: 10g

- Fiber: 7g

- Sugars: 2g

Greek Yogurt and Berry Parfait

Prep Time: 5 mins

Total Time: 5 mins

Servings: 1 parfait

Ingredients:

- 1 cup Greek yogurt
- 1/2 cup mixed berries (blueberries, raspberries)
- 2 tablespoons chopped walnuts
- 1 tablespoon honey
- 1/4 teaspoon vanilla extract

Directions:

1. In a glass, layer Greek yogurt, mixed berries, and chopped walnuts.
2. Drizzle honey over each layer.
3. Repeat the layers until the glass is filled.
4. Finish with a dash of vanilla extract on top.

Nutritional Information (per serving):

- Calories: 290
- Protein: 17g
- Fat: 16g
- Carbohydrates: 22g
- Fiber: 3g
- Sugars: 17g

SNACKS RECIPES

Turmeric Roasted Chickpeas

Prep Time: 5 mins

Total Time: 25 mins

Servings: 4 servings

Ingredients:

- 2 cans (15 oz. each) chickpeas, drained and rinsed
- 2 tablespoons olive oil
- 1 teaspoon ground turmeric
- 1/2 teaspoon cayenne pepper
- 1/2 teaspoon cumin
- Salt to taste

Directions:

1. Preheat the oven to 400°F (200°C).
2. In a bowl, toss chickpeas with olive oil, turmeric, cayenne pepper, cumin, and salt.
3. Spread chickpeas on a baking sheet in a single layer.
4. Roast for 20-25 minutes, shaking the pan halfway through, until golden and crispy.
5. Let them cool before serving.

Nutritional Information (per serving):

- Calories: 180
- Protein: 7g
- Fat: 7g
- Carbohydrates: 24g

- Fiber: 7g

- Sugars: 4g

Avocado and Tomato Salsa

Prep Time: 10 mins

Total Time: 10 mins

Servings: 4 servings

Ingredients:

- 2 ripe avocados, diced

- 1 cup cherry tomatoes, halved

- 1/4 cup red onion, finely chopped

- 1/4 cup fresh cilantro, chopped

- 1 lime, juiced

- Salt and pepper to taste

- Whole-grain crackers for serving

Directions:

1. In a bowl, combine diced avocados, cherry tomatoes, red onion, and cilantro.

2. Drizzle lime juice over the mixture and toss gently.

3. Season with salt and pepper to taste.

4. Serve with whole-grain crackers.

Nutritional Information (per serving):

- Calories: 120

- Protein: 2g

- Fat: 10g

- Carbohydrates: 8g

- Fiber: 5g

- Sugars: 1g

Greek Yogurt and Berry Popsicles

Prep Time: 10 mins

Total Time: 4 hours (including freezing time)

Servings: 6 popsicles

Ingredients:

- 2 cups Greek yogurt
- 1 cup mixed berries (blueberries, strawberries)
- 2 tablespoons honey
- 1 teaspoon vanilla extract

Directions:

1. In a bowl, mix Greek yogurt, mixed berries, honey, and vanilla extract.
2. Spoon the mixture into popsicle molds.
3. Insert popsicle sticks and freeze for at least 4 hours or overnight.
4. Run molds under warm water to release the popsicles.

Nutritional Information (per serving):

- Calories: 100
- Protein: 7g
- Fat: 2g
- Carbohydrates: 15g
- Fiber: 1g
- Sugars: 12g

Almond Butter and Banana Energy Bites

Prep Time: 15 mins

Total Time: 15 mins

Servings: 12 bites

Ingredients:

- 1 cup rolled oats
- 1/2 cup almond butter
- 1/4 cup honey
- 1/2 cup mashed banana
- 1/4 cup chopped almonds
- 1/4 cup chia seeds
- 1/2 teaspoon cinnamon

Directions:

1. In a bowl, combine rolled oats, almond butter, honey, mashed banana, chopped almonds, chia seeds, and cinnamon.
2. Mix until well combined.
3. Roll the mixture into bite-sized balls and place on a lined tray.
4. Refrigerate for at least 1 hour before serving.

Nutritional Information (per serving - 2 bites):

- Calories: 180
- Protein: 5g
- Fat: 9g
- Carbohydrates: 23g
- Fiber: 4g
- Sugars: 9g

Veggie and Hummus Stuffed Cucumber Bites

Prep Time: 15 mins

Total Time: 15 mins

Servings: 4 servings

Ingredients:

- 2 cucumbers, sliced into rounds
- 1 cup hummus
- 1 cup cherry tomatoes, quartered
- 1/2 cup cucumber, diced
- 1/4 cup red onion, finely chopped
- Fresh dill for garnish

Directions:

1. Using a spoon, hollow out the center of each cucumber round to create a cup.
2. Fill each cucumber cup with hummus.
3. Top with cherry tomatoes, diced cucumber, and red onion.
4. Garnish with fresh dill before serving.

Nutritional Information (per serving):

- Calories: 160
- Protein: 6g
- Fat: 8g
- Carbohydrates: 18g
- Fiber: 6g
- Sugars: 5g

Spiced Almond and Pumpkin Seed Mix

Prep Time: 5 mins

Total Time: 10 mins

Servings: 4 servings

Ingredients:

- 1 cup raw almonds
- 1/2 cup pumpkin seeds
- 1 tablespoon olive oil
- 1/2 teaspoon ground cumin
- 1/2 teaspoon smoked paprika
- 1/4 teaspoon cayenne pepper
- Salt to taste

Directions:

1. In a pan, heat olive oil over medium heat.
2. Add almonds and pumpkin seeds, tossing until lightly toasted.
3. Sprinkle cumin, smoked paprika, cayenne pepper, and salt over the nuts.
4. Continue toasting for an additional 2-3 minutes.
5. Let the mixture cool before serving.

Nutritional Information (per serving):

- Calories: 210
- Protein: 8g
- Fat: 18g
- Carbohydrates: 7g
- Fiber: 4g
- Sugars: 1g

Stuffed Bell Pepper Poppers

Prep Time: 15 mins

Total Time: 30 mins

Servings: 6 servings

Ingredients:

- 3 bell peppers, halved and seeds removed
- 1 cup hummus
- 1 cup cherry tomatoes, quartered
- 1/2 cup cucumber, diced
- 1/4 cup red onion, finely chopped
- Fresh parsley for garnish

Directions:

1. Preheat the oven to 375°F (190°C).
2. Fill each bell pepper half with hummus.
3. Top with cherry tomatoes, cucumber, and red onion.
4. Place the stuffed peppers on a baking sheet and bake for 15-20 minutes.
5. Garnish with fresh parsley before serving.

Nutritional Information (per serving):

- Calories: 120
- Protein: 4g
- Fat: 7g
- Carbohydrates: 12g
- Fiber: 4g
- Sugars: 2g

Mango and Avocado Salsa with Whole-Grain Chips

Prep Time: 10 mins

Total Time: 10 mins

Servings: 4 servings

Ingredients:

- 1 ripe mango, diced
- 1 avocado, diced
- 1/4 cup red onion, finely chopped
- 1/4 cup fresh cilantro, chopped
- 1 lime, juiced
- Salt and pepper to taste
- Whole-grain tortilla chips for serving

Directions:

1. In a bowl, combine diced mango, avocado, red onion, and cilantro.
2. Drizzle lime juice over the mixture and toss gently.
3. Season with salt and pepper to taste.
4. Serve with whole-grain tortilla chips.

Nutritional Information (per serving):

- Calories: 150
- Protein: 2g
- Fat: 10g
- Carbohydrates: 18g
- Fiber: 5g
- Sugars: 8g

Baked Sweet Potato Fries with Rosemary

Prep Time: 10 mins

Total Time: 30 mins

Servings: 3 servings

Ingredients:

- 2 large sweet potatoes, cut into fries
- 2 tablespoons olive oil
- 1 tablespoon fresh rosemary, chopped
- Salt and pepper to taste

Directions:

1. Preheat the oven to 425°F (220°C).
2. In a bowl, toss sweet potato fries with olive oil, rosemary, salt, and pepper.
3. Spread the fries in a single layer on a baking sheet.
4. Bake for 20-25 minutes, turning halfway through, until crispy.
5. Let them cool slightly before serving.

Nutritional Information (per serving):

- Calories: 180
- Protein: 2g
- Fat: 7g
- Carbohydrates: 29g
- Fiber: 4g
- Sugars: 5g

Protein-Packed Yogurt Parfait

Prep Time: 10 mins

Total Time: 10 mins

Servings: 2 parfaits

Ingredients:

- 1 cup Greek yogurt
- 1/2 cup granola (choose a low-sugar option)
- 1/2 cup mixed berries (blueberries, strawberries)
- 2 tablespoons chopped nuts (almonds, walnuts)
- 1 tablespoon honey

Directions:

1. In a glass or bowl, layer Greek yogurt, granola, mixed berries, and chopped nuts.
2. Drizzle honey over each layer.
3. Repeat the layers until the glass is filled.
4. Enjoy immediately.

Nutritional Information (per serving):

- Calories: 280
- Protein: 15g
- Fat: 10g
- Carbohydrates: 30g
- Fiber: 4g
- Sugars: 16g

Crispy Kale Chips with Sea Salt

Prep Time: 10 mins

Total Time: 20 mins

Servings: 4 servings

Ingredients:

- 1 bunch kale, stems removed and torn into bite-sized pieces
- 2 tablespoons olive oil

- Sea salt to taste

Directions:

1. Preheat the oven to 350°F (175°C).
2. In a bowl, massage kale pieces with olive oil until well coated.
3. Spread kale on a baking sheet in a single layer.
4. Sprinkle with sea salt.
5. Bake for 10-15 minutes until crispy, checking regularly to avoid burning.
6. Allow to cool before serving.

Nutritional Information (per serving):

- Calories: 80
- Protein: 3g
- Fat: 5g
- Carbohydrates: 8g
- Fiber: 2g
- Sugars: 1g

Quinoa and Veggie Stuffed Mushrooms

Prep Time: 15 mins

Total Time: 30 mins

Servings: 6 servings

Ingredients:

- 12 large mushrooms, stems removed
- 1 cup cooked quinoa
- 1/2 cup bell peppers, diced
- 1/4 cup red onion, finely chopped
- 1/4 cup cherry tomatoes, quartered

- 2 tablespoons olive oil
- 1 teaspoon Italian seasoning
- Salt and pepper to taste

Directions:

1. Preheat the oven to 375°F (190°C).
2. In a bowl, mix cooked quinoa, bell peppers, red onion, cherry tomatoes, olive oil, Italian seasoning, salt, and pepper.
3. Stuff each mushroom cap with the quinoa mixture.
4. Place stuffed mushrooms on a baking sheet and bake for 15-20 minutes.
5. Allow to cool slightly before serving.

Nutritional Information (per serving):

- Calories: 120
- Protein: 4g
- Fat: 7g
- Carbohydrates: 13g
- Fiber: 2g
- Sugars: 2g

Sesame Ginger Edamame

Prep Time: 5 mins

Total Time: 10 mins

Servings: 4 servings

Ingredients:

- 2 cups frozen edamame, thawed
- 1 tablespoon sesame oil
- 1 tablespoon soy sauce

- 1 teaspoon fresh ginger, grated
- 1 teaspoon sesame seeds

Directions:

1. In a pan, heat sesame oil over medium heat.
2. Add thawed edamame, soy sauce, and grated ginger.
3. Sauté for 5-7 minutes until heated through.
4. Sprinkle with sesame seeds before serving.

Nutritional Information (per serving):

- Calories: 120
- Protein: 9g
- Fat: 6g
- Carbohydrates: 8g
- Fiber: 4g
- Sugars: 2g

Cucumber Roll-Ups with Hummus and Turkey

Prep Time: 15 mins

Total Time: 15 mins

Servings: 4 servings

Ingredients:

- 2 large cucumbers, thinly sliced lengthwise
- 1/2 cup hummus
- 1/2 pound smoked turkey, thinly sliced
- Fresh dill for garnish

Directions:

1. Lay cucumber slices flat and spread a thin layer of hummus on each.

2. Place a slice of turkey on top of each cucumber slice.

3. Roll up each slice and secure with a toothpick.

4. Garnish with fresh dill before serving.

Nutritional Information (per serving):

- Calories: 140
- Protein: 12g
- Fat: 6g
- Carbohydrates: 10g
- Fiber: 3g
- Sugars: 4g

Baked Apple Chips

Prep Time: 10 mins

Total Time: 2 hours

Servings: 4 servings

Ingredients:

- 2 large apples, thinly sliced
- 1 tablespoon cinnamon
- 1 tablespoon honey (optional)

Directions:

1. Preheat the oven to 200°F (95°C).

2. In a bowl, toss apple slices with cinnamon and honey (if using).

3. Place the slices on a baking sheet in a single layer.

4. Bake for 2 hours, flipping halfway through.

5. Let them cool before serving.

Nutritional Information (per serving):

- Calories: 90

- Protein: 0.5g

- Fat: 0.3g

- Carbohydrates: 24g

- Fiber: 4g

- Sugars: 18g

Baked Sweet Potato Chips

Prep Time: 10 mins

Total Time: 25 mins

Servings: 4 servings

Ingredients:

- 2 medium sweet potatoes, thinly sliced

- 2 tablespoons olive oil

- 1/2 teaspoon paprika

- 1/2 teaspoon garlic powder

- Salt to taste

Directions:

1. Preheat the oven to 400°F (200°C).

2. In a bowl, toss sweet potato slices with olive oil, paprika, garlic powder, and salt.

3. Arrange slices on a baking sheet in a single layer.

4. Bake for 15-20 minutes, flipping halfway through, until crispy.

5. Allow to cool before serving.

Nutritional Information (per serving):

- Calories: 120

- Protein: 2g

- Fat: 5g

- Carbohydrates: 20g

- Fiber: 4g

- Sugars: 5g

Salmon and Avocado Nori Rolls

Prep Time: 15 mins

Total Time: 15 mins

Servings: 4 servings

Ingredients:

- 4 sheets nori seaweed

- 1 cup cooked quinoa

- 2 ounces smoked salmon

- 1 avocado, sliced

- 1/2 cucumber, julienned

- Soy sauce for dipping

Directions:

1. Place a nori sheet on a bamboo sushi rolling mat.

2. Spread a thin layer of quinoa over the nori.

3. Arrange smoked salmon, avocado, and cucumber along one edge.

4. Roll tightly and slice into bite-sized pieces.

5. Serve with soy sauce for dipping.

Nutritional Information (per serving):

- Calories: 180

- Protein: 8g

- Fat: 8g

- Carbohydrates: 20g

- Fiber: 5g

- Sugars: 1g

Roasted Red Pepper Hummus with Veggie Sticks

Prep Time: 10 mins

Total Time: 15 mins

Servings: 4 servings

Ingredients:

- 1 cup chickpeas, drained and rinsed

- 1/2 cup roasted red peppers

- 2 tablespoons tahini

- 1 garlic clove

- 2 tablespoons olive oil

- Assorted vegetable sticks (carrots, bell peppers, cucumber)

Directions:

1. In a food processor, blend chickpeas, roasted red peppers, tahini, garlic, and olive oil until smooth.

2. Serve hummus with assorted vegetable sticks.

Nutritional Information (per serving):

- Calories: 150

- Protein: 5g

- Fat: 10g

- Carbohydrates: 13g

- Fiber: 4g

- Sugars: 2g

Greek Yogurt and Berry Parfait

Prep Time: 10 mins

Total Time: 10 mins

Servings: 2 servings

Ingredients:

- 1 cup Greek yogurt
- 1/2 cup mixed berries (blueberries, strawberries)
- 1/4 cup granola (choose a low-sugar option)
- 1 tablespoon honey

Directions:

1. In a glass or bowl, layer Greek yogurt, mixed berries, and granola.
2. Drizzle honey over each layer.
3. Repeat the layers until the glass is filled.
4. Enjoy immediately.

Nutritional Information (per serving):

- Calories: 250
- Protein: 15g
- Fat: 8g
- Carbohydrates: 30g
- Fiber: 3g
- Sugars: 18g

Chia Seed Pudding with Mango

Prep Time: 5 mins (plus overnight chilling)

Total Time: 5 mins (plus overnight chilling)

Servings: 2 servings

Ingredients:

- 1/4 cup chia seeds
- 1 cup almond milk
- 1 teaspoon vanilla extract
- 1 tablespoon honey
- 1 ripe mango, diced

Directions:

1. In a bowl, whisk together chia seeds, almond milk, vanilla extract, and honey.
2. Cover and refrigerate overnight.
3. Before serving, stir well and top with diced mango.

Nutritional Information (per serving):

- Calories: 180
- Protein: 4g
- Fat: 7g
- Carbohydrates: 27g
- Fiber: 8g
- Sugars: 15g

DESSERTS RECIPES

Baked Apple Cinnamon Oat Cups

Prep Time: 15 mins

Total Time: 40 mins

Servings: 6 servings

Ingredients:

- 2 cups old-fashioned oats
- 1 cup unsweetened applesauce
- 1/4 cup honey or maple syrup
- 1 teaspoon ground cinnamon
- 1/2 teaspoon vanilla extract
- 1/2 cup chopped walnuts
- 2 medium apples, peeled and diced

Directions:

1. Preheat the oven to 350°F (175°C).
2. In a bowl, mix oats, applesauce, honey, cinnamon, vanilla extract, walnuts, and diced apples.
3. Divide the mixture into greased muffin cups.
4. Bake for 25-30 minutes until golden brown.
5. Allow to cool before serving.

Nutritional Information (per serving):

- Calories: 220
- Protein: 4g
- Fat: 8g
- Carbohydrates: 35g

- Fiber: 5g

- Sugars: 16g

Dark Chocolate Avocado Mousse

Prep Time: 10 mins

Total Time: 2 hours (including chilling time)

Servings: 4 servings

Ingredients:

- 2 ripe avocados

- 1/2 cup unsweetened cocoa powder

- 1/4 cup honey or agave nectar

- 1 teaspoon vanilla extract

- A pinch of sea salt

- Dark chocolate shavings for garnish (optional)

Directions:

1. In a blender, combine avocados, cocoa powder, honey, vanilla extract, and salt.

2. Blend until smooth and creamy.

3. Refrigerate for at least 2 hours.

4. Spoon into serving dishes and garnish with dark chocolate shavings if desired.

Nutritional Information (per serving):

- Calories: 220

- Protein: 4g

- Fat: 14g

- Carbohydrates: 26g

- Fiber: 9g

- Sugars: 13g

Berry Almond Chia Pudding

Prep Time: 10 mins

Total Time: 2 hours (including chilling time)

Servings: 4 servings

Ingredients:

- 1/2 cup chia seeds
- 2 cups almond milk
- 1 teaspoon vanilla extract
- 1 tablespoon honey
- 1 cup mixed berries (blueberries, strawberries, raspberries)
- Sliced almonds for garnish

Directions:

1. In a bowl, whisk together chia seeds, almond milk, vanilla extract, and honey.
2. Refrigerate for at least 2 hours or overnight.
3. Before serving, stir well and top with mixed berries and sliced almonds.

Nutritional Information (per serving):

- Calories: 180
- Protein: 5g
- Fat: 9g
- Carbohydrates: 23g
- Fiber: 9g
- Sugars: 8g

Peach and Coconut Sorbet

Prep Time: 10 mins

Total Time: 4 hours (including freezing time)

Servings: 4 servings

Ingredients:

- 4 ripe peaches, peeled and sliced
- 1 can (13.5 oz.) coconut milk
- 1/4 cup honey or agave nectar
- 1 tablespoon lemon juice

Directions:

1. In a blender, combine sliced peaches, coconut milk, honey, and lemon juice.
2. Blend until smooth.
3. Pour the mixture into a shallow dish and freeze for at least 4 hours, stirring every hour.
4. Scoop and serve when the sorbet reaches the desired consistency.

Nutritional Information (per serving):

- Calories: 180
- Protein: 2g
- Fat: 10g
- Carbohydrates: 22g
- Fiber: 3g
- Sugars: 18g

Cherry Almond Energy Bites

Prep Time: 15 mins

Total Time: 30 mins

Servings: 12 servings

Ingredients:

- 1 cup dried cherries
- 1 cup almonds
- 1/2 cup rolled oats
- 1/4 cup almond butter
- 1/4 cup honey
- 1 teaspoon vanilla extract
- Pinch of sea salt

Directions:

1. In a food processor, pulse dried cherries, almonds, and rolled oats until finely chopped.
2. Add almond butter, honey, vanilla extract, and a pinch of sea salt.
3. Pulse until the mixture comes together.
4. Roll into bite-sized balls and refrigerate for 15 minutes before serving.

Nutritional Information (per serving):

- Calories: 140
- Protein: 4g
- Fat: 8g
- Carbohydrates: 16g
- Fiber: 3g
- Sugars: 9g

Guilt-Free Mango Sorbet

Prep Time: 10 mins

Total Time: 4 hours (including freezing time)

Servings: 4 servings

Ingredients:

- 2 cups frozen mango chunks
- 1/4 cup coconut water
- 1 tablespoon lime juice
- 1 tablespoon agave nectar or honey
- Fresh mint leaves for garnish

Directions:

1. In a blender, combine frozen mango chunks, coconut water, lime juice, and agave nectar.
2. Blend until smooth.
3. Pour the mixture into a shallow dish and freeze for at least 4 hours, stirring every hour.
4. Scoop into bowls, garnish with fresh mint leaves, and serve.

Nutritional Information (per serving):

- Calories: 90
- Protein: 1g
- Fat: 0.5g
- Carbohydrates: 23g
- Fiber: 2g
- Sugars: 20g

Chia Seed Chocolate Pudding

Prep Time: 10 mins

Total Time: 2 hours (including chilling time)

Servings: 4 servings

Ingredients:

- 1/4 cup chia seeds
- 2 cups unsweetened almond milk
- 2 tablespoons unsweetened cocoa powder
- 2 tablespoons maple syrup
- 1 teaspoon vanilla extract
- Fresh berries for topping

Directions:

1. In a bowl, whisk together chia seeds, almond milk, cocoa powder, maple syrup, and vanilla extract.
2. Refrigerate for at least 2 hours or overnight.
3. Stir well before serving and top with fresh berries.

Nutritional Information (per serving):

- Calories: 120
- Protein: 3g
- Fat: 6g
- Carbohydrates: 16g
- Fiber: 6g
- Sugars: 6g

Baked Almond Berry Crisp

Prep Time: 15 mins

Total Time: 45 mins

Servings: 6 servings

Ingredients:

- 3 cups mixed berries (strawberries, blueberries, raspberries)
- 1 tablespoon lemon juice
- 1/4 cup honey or agave nectar
- 1 cup almond flour
- 1/4 cup coconut oil, melted
- 1/2 cup sliced almonds

Directions:

1. Preheat the oven to 350°F (175°C).
2. In a bowl, toss mixed berries with lemon juice and honey.
3. Transfer the berries to a baking dish.
4. In another bowl, combine almond flour, melted coconut oil, and sliced almonds.
5. Crumble the almond mixture over the berries.
6. Bake for 30-35 minutes until the top is golden brown.
7. Allow to cool slightly before serving.

Nutritional Information (per serving):

- Calories: 250
- Protein: 5g
- Fat: 18g
- Carbohydrates: 21g
- Fiber: 6g
- Sugars: 12g

Pineapple Coconut Nice Cream

Prep Time: 10 mins

Total Time: 4 hours (including freezing time)

Servings: 4 servings

Ingredients:

- 2 cups frozen pineapple chunks
- 1/2 cup coconut milk
- 1 tablespoon shredded coconut
- 1 tablespoon honey or agave nectar
- Toasted coconut flakes for garnish

Directions:

1. In a blender, blend frozen pineapple chunks, coconut milk, shredded coconut, and honey until creamy.
2. Pour the mixture into a shallow dish and freeze for at least 4 hours, stirring every hour.
3. Serve in bowls, garnished with toasted coconut flakes.

Nutritional Information (per serving):

- Calories: 120
- Protein: 1g
- Fat: 5g
- Carbohydrates: 20g
- Fiber: 2g
- Sugars: 16g

Banana Walnut Bites

Prep Time: 15 mins

Total Time: 30 mins

Servings: 12 servings

Ingredients:

- 3 ripe bananas, mashed
- 1/2 cup chopped walnuts
- 1/4 cup coconut flour
- 1/4 cup almond butter
- 1 teaspoon vanilla extract
- 1/2 teaspoon cinnamon
- Pinch of sea salt

Directions:

1. Preheat the oven to 350°F (175°C).
2. In a bowl, mix mashed bananas, chopped walnuts, coconut flour, almond butter, vanilla extract, cinnamon, and a pinch of sea salt.
3. Drop spoonfuls of the mixture onto a baking sheet.
4. Bake for 15-20 minutes until golden brown.
5. Allow to cool before serving.

Nutritional Information (per serving):

- Calories: 90
- Protein: 2g
- Fat: 5g
- Carbohydrates: 11g
- Fiber: 2g
- Sugars: 5g

Ginger Turmeric Golden Milk Popsicles

Prep Time: 10 mins

Total Time: 4 hours (including freezing time)

Servings: 6 popsicles

Ingredients:

- 2 cups coconut milk
- 1 teaspoon ground turmeric
- 1 teaspoon ground ginger
- 2 tablespoons honey
- 1/2 teaspoon vanilla extract
- Pinch of black pepper (enhances turmeric absorption)

Directions:

1. In a saucepan, heat coconut milk, turmeric, ginger, honey, vanilla extract, and black pepper.
2. Whisk until well combined and heated through.
3. Allow the mixture to cool, then pour into popsicle molds.
4. Freeze for at least 4 hours before enjoying.

Nutritional Information (per serving):

- Calories: 90
- Protein: 1g
- Fat: 7g
- Carbohydrates: 6g
- Fiber: 0.5g
- Sugars: 4g

Chia Seed Chocolate Pudding

Prep Time: 10 mins

Total Time: 2 hours (including chilling time)

Servings: 4 servings

Ingredients:

- 1/2 cup chia seeds
- 2 cups almond milk
- 3 tablespoons unsweetened cocoa powder
- 2 tablespoons maple syrup
- 1 teaspoon vanilla extract
- Fresh berries for garnish

Directions:

1. In a bowl, whisk together chia seeds, almond milk, cocoa powder, maple syrup, and vanilla extract.
2. Refrigerate for at least 2 hours or overnight.
3. Stir well before serving and garnish with fresh berries.

Nutritional Information (per serving):

- Calories: 180
- Protein: 5g
- Fat: 9g
- Carbohydrates: 23g
- Fiber: 9g
- Sugars: 7g

Mango Coconut Rice Pudding

Prep Time: 15 mins

Total Time: 45 mins

Servings: 4 servings

Ingredients:

- 1 cup cooked brown rice
- 1 cup coconut milk
- 1 ripe mango, diced
- 2 tablespoons honey or agave nectar
- 1/2 teaspoon ground cinnamon
- Sliced almonds for garnish

Directions:

1. In a saucepan, combine brown rice, coconut milk, diced mango, honey, and cinnamon.
2. Cook over medium heat until the mixture thickens, stirring occasionally.
3. Remove from heat and let it cool.
4. Serve topped with sliced almonds.

Nutritional Information (per serving):

- Calories: 230
- Protein: 4g
- Fat: 8g
- Carbohydrates: 36g
- Fiber: 3g
- Sugars: 15g

Almond Butter Banana Bites

Prep Time: 10 mins

Total Time: 20 mins

Servings: 8 servings

Ingredients:

- 2 large bananas, peeled and sliced
- 1/4 cup almond butter
- 1/4 cup unsweetened shredded coconut
- 2 tablespoons chopped almonds

Directions:

1. Spread almond butter on banana slices.
2. Roll the edges in shredded coconut and chopped almonds.
3. Place on a parchment-lined tray and freeze for 10 minutes.
4. Serve immediately.

Nutritional Information (per serving):

- Calories: 90
- Protein: 2g
- Fat: 6g
- Carbohydrates: 9g
- Fiber: 2g
- Sugars: 4g

Cinnamon Baked Pears

Prep Time: 10 mins

Total Time: 30 mins

Servings: 4 servings

Ingredients:

- 2 ripe pears, halved and cored
- 1 tablespoon melted coconut oil
- 1 teaspoon ground cinnamon
- 2 tablespoons chopped walnuts
- Greek yogurt for serving

Directions:

1. Preheat the oven to 375°F (190°C).
2. Place pear halves on a baking sheet.
3. Brush with melted coconut oil and sprinkle with cinnamon.
4. Bake for 20-25 minutes until tender.
5. Sprinkle with chopped walnuts and serve with a dollop of Greek yogurt.

Nutritional Information (per serving):

- Calories: 120
- Protein: 2g
- Fat: 7g
- Carbohydrates: 15g
- Fiber: 4g
- Sugars: 8g

Blueberry Chia Seed Pudding Parfait

Prep Time: 10 mins

Total Time: 2 hours (including chilling time)

Servings: 4 servings

Ingredients:

- 1 cup blueberries
- 1/2 cup chia seeds
- 2 cups almond milk
- 2 tablespoons honey or maple syrup
- 1 teaspoon vanilla extract
- Granola for layering

Directions:

1. In a blender, mix blueberries, chia seeds, almond milk, honey, and vanilla extract until smooth.

2. Refrigerate the mixture for at least 2 hours or overnight.

3. In serving glasses, layer the chia pudding with granola.

4. Repeat layers and top with additional blueberries.

Nutritional Information (per serving):

- Calories: 180
- Protein: 5g
- Fat: 8g
- Carbohydrates: 24g
- Fiber: 8g
- Sugars: 12g

Turmeric Mango Sorbet

Prep Time: 15 mins

Total Time: 4 hours (including freezing time)

Servings: 4 servings

Ingredients:

- 2 ripe mangoes, peeled and diced
- 1 can (13.5 oz) coconut milk
- 1 tablespoon honey or agave nectar
- 1 teaspoon ground turmeric
- 1 tablespoon fresh lime juice

Directions:

1. In a blender, combine diced mangoes, coconut milk, honey, turmeric, and lime juice.

2. Blend until smooth.

3. Pour the mixture into a shallow dish and freeze for at least 4 hours, stirring every hour.

4. Serve when the sorbet reaches the desired consistency.

Nutritional Information (per serving):

- Calories: 220
- Protein: 2g
- Fat: 14g
- Carbohydrates: 24g
- Fiber: 3g
- Sugars: 18g

Pineapple Mint Frozen Yogurt

Prep Time: 10 mins

Total Time: 2 hours (including freezing time)

Servings: 4 servings

Ingredients:

- 2 cups frozen pineapple chunks
- 1 cup Greek yogurt
- 2 tablespoons honey
- Fresh mint leaves for garnish

Directions:

1. In a food processor, blend frozen pineapple chunks, Greek yogurt, and honey until smooth.

2. Transfer the mixture to a container and freeze for at least 2 hours.

3. Scoop and garnish with fresh mint leaves before serving.

Nutritional Information (per serving):

- Calories: 120

- Protein: 8g

- Fat: 0.5g

- Carbohydrates: 26g

- Fiber: 2g

- Sugars: 21g

Chocolate Avocado Mousse with Berries

Prep Time: 15 mins

Total Time: 2 hours (including chilling time)

Servings: 4 servings

Ingredients:

- 2 ripe avocados

- 1/4 cup cocoa powder

- 1/4 cup honey or agave nectar

- 1 teaspoon vanilla extract

- Mixed berries for topping

Directions:

1. In a blender, combine avocados, cocoa powder, honey, and vanilla extract.

2. Blend until smooth and creamy.

3. Refrigerate for at least 2 hours.

4. Spoon into serving dishes and top with mixed berries.

Nutritional Information (per serving):

- Calories: 180

- Protein: 3g

- Fat: 11g

- Carbohydrates: 24g

- Fiber: 7g

- Sugars: 15g

Almond Butter Banana Ice Cream

Prep Time: 5 mins

Total Time: 4 hours (including freezing time)

Servings: 4 servings

Ingredients:

- 4 ripe bananas, sliced and frozen

- 1/4 cup almond butter

- 1/4 cup unsweetened almond milk

- 1 tablespoon honey or maple syrup

- Sliced almonds for topping

Directions:

1. In a blender, combine frozen banana slices, almond butter, almond milk, and honey.

2. Blend until smooth and creamy.

3. Transfer the mixture to a container and freeze for at least 4 hours.

4. Serve topped with sliced almonds.

Nutritional Information (per serving):

- Calories: 190

- Protein: 3g

- Fat: 7g

- Carbohydrates: 31g

- Fiber: 4g

- Sugars: 16g

BEVERAGES RECIPES

Anti-Inflammatory Turmeric Tea

Prep Time: 5 mins

Total Time: 10 mins

Servings: 2 cups

Ingredients:

- 2 cups water
- 1 teaspoon ground turmeric
- 1/2 teaspoon ground ginger
- 1 tablespoon honey
- 1/2 lemon, juiced
- Pinch of black pepper

Directions:

1. In a saucepan, bring water to a boil.
2. Add turmeric, ginger, honey, lemon juice, and a pinch of black pepper.
3. Simmer for 5 minutes.
4. Strain into cups and enjoy the soothing effects.

Nutritional Information (per serving):

- Calories: 30
- Protein: 0.5g
- Fat: 0g
- Carbohydrates: 8g
- Fiber: 1g
- Sugars: 6g

Green Goddess Smoothie

Prep Time: 10 mins

Total Time: 5 mins

Servings: 2 glasses

Ingredients:

- 1 cup frozen pineapple chunks
- 1/2 cucumber, peeled and sliced
- 1 cup kale leaves, stems removed
- 1/2 avocado
- 1 tablespoon chia seeds
- 1 cup coconut water
- Ice cubes (optional)

Directions:

1. In a blender, combine frozen pineapple, cucumber, kale, avocado, chia seeds, and coconut water.
2. Blend until smooth.
3. Add ice cubes if a colder temperature is desired.
4. Pour into glasses and savor the refreshing taste.

Nutritional Information (per serving):

- Calories: 150
- Protein: 4g
- Fat: 8g
- Carbohydrates: 19g
- Fiber: 8g
- Sugars: 8g

Berry Blast Arthritis Smoothie

Prep Time: 8 mins

Total Time: 3 mins

Servings: 2 glasses

Ingredients:

- 1 cup mixed berries (blueberries, strawberries, raspberries)
- 1/2 cup Greek yogurt
- 1 cup almond milk
- 1 tablespoon flaxseeds
- 1 tablespoon honey
- Ice cubes (optional)

Directions:

1. Combine mixed berries, Greek yogurt, almond milk, flaxseeds, and honey in a blender.
2. Blend until smooth.
3. Add ice cubes if desired for a colder consistency.
4. Pour into glasses and relish the fruity goodness.

Nutritional Information (per serving):

- Calories: 180
- Protein: 8g
- Fat: 6g
- Carbohydrates: 25g
- Fiber: 7g
- Sugars: 15g

Cucumber Mint Infused Water

Prep Time: 5 mins

Total Time: 1 hour (infusing time)

Servings: 2 glasses

Ingredients:

- 2 cups water
- 1/2 cucumber, thinly sliced
- Handful of fresh mint leaves
- Ice cubes (optional)

Directions:

1. In a pitcher, combine water, cucumber slices, and mint leaves.
2. Refrigerate for at least 1 hour to infuse flavors.
3. Add ice cubes if desired.
4. Pour into glasses and enjoy the hydrating infusion.

Nutritional Information (per serving):

- Calories: 0
- Protein: 0g
- Fat: 0g
- Carbohydrates: 0g
- Fiber: 0g
- Sugars: 0g

Golden Almond Milk Latte

Prep Time: 5 mins

Total Time: 10 mins

Servings: 2 cups

Ingredients:

- 2 cups almond milk

- 1 teaspoon ground turmeric

- 1/2 teaspoon cinnamon

- 1 tablespoon honey

- 1 teaspoon vanilla extract

Directions:

1. In a saucepan, heat almond milk, turmeric, cinnamon, honey, and vanilla extract.

2. Whisk until well combined and warmed.

3. Pour into cups and savor the comforting golden latte.

Nutritional Information (per serving):

- Calories: 80

- Protein: 1g

- Fat: 4g

- Carbohydrates: 10g

- Fiber: 1g

- Sugars: 7g

Tropical Pineapple Ginger Smoothie

Prep Time: 8 mins

Total Time: 3 mins

Servings: 2 glasses

Ingredients:

- 1 cup frozen pineapple chunks

- 1/2-inch fresh ginger, peeled and chopped

- 1 cup coconut water

- 1/2 banana

- Handful of fresh mint leaves

* 1 tablespoon chia seeds

Directions:

1. In a blender, combine frozen pineapple, fresh ginger, coconut water, banana, mint leaves, and chia seeds.

2. Blend until smooth.

3. Pour into glasses and enjoy the tropical refreshment.

Nutritional Information (per serving):

* Calories: 120

* Protein: 3g

* Fat: 2g

* Carbohydrates: 26g

* Fiber: 5g

* Sugars: 15g

Berry Citrus Hydration Drink

Prep Time: 5 mins

Total Time: 2 mins

Servings: 2 glasses

Ingredients:

* 1 cup mixed berries (strawberries, blueberries, raspberries)

* 1 orange, peeled and segmented

* 2 cups water

* 1 tablespoon honey

* Ice cubes (optional)

Directions:

1. In a blender, combine mixed berries, orange segments, water, and honey.

2. Blend until well combined.

3. Strain if desired and pour into glasses.

4. Add ice cubes for a cooler drink.

Nutritional Information (per serving):

- Calories: 80
- Protein: 1g
- Fat: 0.5g
- Carbohydrates: 20g
- Fiber: 5g
- Sugars: 14g

Minty Cucumber Lemonade

Prep Time: 10 mins

Total Time: 5 mins

Servings: 2 glasses

Ingredients:

- 1 cucumber, thinly sliced
- 1 lemon, juiced
- Handful of fresh mint leaves
- 2 cups water
- 1 tablespoon agave nectar or honey
- Lemon slices for garnish

Directions:

1. In a pitcher, combine cucumber slices, lemon juice, mint leaves, water, and agave nectar.

2. Stir well to mix flavors.

3. Pour into glasses over ice.

4. Garnish with lemon slices.

Nutritional Information (per serving):

- Calories: 40
- Protein: 1g
- Fat: 0g
- Carbohydrates: 10g
- Fiber: 2g
- Sugars: 6g

Golden Turmeric Iced Tea

Prep Time: 5 mins

Total Time: 15 mins

Servings: 2 glasses

Ingredients:

- 2 cups brewed green tea, cooled
- 1/2 teaspoon ground turmeric
- 1 tablespoon honey
- 1/2 teaspoon lemon zest
- Ice cubes

Directions:

1. In a pitcher, mix brewed green tea, ground turmeric, honey, and lemon zest.
2. Stir until well combined.
3. Refrigerate for at least 10 minutes.
4. Serve over ice.

Nutritional Information (per serving):

- Calories: 20

- Protein: 0g

- Fat: 0g

- Carbohydrates: 5g

- Fiber: 0g

- Sugars: 4g

Coconut Berry Protein Smoothie

Prep Time: 8 mins

Total Time: 3 mins

Servings: 2 glasses

Ingredients:

- 1 cup mixed berries (blueberries, raspberries, blackberries)

- 1 cup coconut water

- 1/2 cup Greek yogurt

- 1 scoop vanilla protein powder

- 1 tablespoon almond butter

- Ice cubes (optional)

Directions:

1. Blend mixed berries, coconut water, Greek yogurt, vanilla protein powder, and almond butter until smooth.

2. Add ice cubes if desired for a colder consistency.

3. Pour into glasses and enjoy the protein-packed goodness.

Nutritional Information (per serving):

- Calories: 180

- Protein: 15g

- Fat: 6g

- Carbohydrates: 18g

- Fiber: 4g

- Sugars: 10g

Mango Turmeric Smoothie

Prep Time: 8 mins

Total Time: 3 mins

Servings: 2 glasses

Ingredients:

- 1 cup frozen mango chunks

- 1/2 teaspoon ground turmeric

- 1 cup almond milk

- 1 tablespoon chia seeds

- 1 tablespoon honey

- 1/2 teaspoon vanilla extract

Directions:

1. In a blender, combine frozen mango, ground turmeric, almond milk, chia seeds, honey, and vanilla extract.

2. Blend until smooth.

3. Pour into glasses and enjoy the tropical goodness.

Nutritional Information (per serving):

- Calories: 150

- Protein: 3g

- Fat: 5g

- Carbohydrates: 25g

- Fiber: 6g

- Sugars: 18g

Cranberry Almond Protein Shake

Prep Time: 5 mins

Total Time: 2 mins

Servings: 2 glasses

Ingredients:

- 1 cup cranberry juice (unsweetened)
- 1/2 cup almond milk
- 1 scoop vanilla protein powder
- 1/4 cup almonds
- 1 tablespoon flaxseeds
- Ice cubes (optional)

Directions:

1. In a blender, combine cranberry juice, almond milk, vanilla protein powder, almonds, and flaxseeds.
2. Blend until well combined.
3. Add ice cubes for a colder shake.
4. Pour into glasses and relish the protein-packed refreshment.

Nutritional Information (per serving):

- Calories: 220
- Protein: 15g
- Fat: 12g
- Carbohydrates: 15g
- Fiber: 4g
- Sugars: 8g

Pineapple Mint Green Tea

Prep Time: 10 mins

Total Time: 5 mins

Servings: 2 glasses

Ingredients:

- 2 cups brewed green tea, cooled
- 1 cup fresh pineapple chunks
- Handful of fresh mint leaves
- 1 tablespoon honey
- Ice cubes

Directions:

1. In a blender, combine brewed green tea, pineapple chunks, mint leaves, and honey.
2. Blend until smooth.
3. Serve over ice and enjoy the refreshing green tea infusion.

Nutritional Information (per serving):

- Calories: 40
- Protein: 0g
- Fat: 0g
- Carbohydrates: 10g
- Fiber: 1g
- Sugars: 8g

Blueberry Avocado Bliss

Prep Time: 8 mins

Total Time: 3 mins

Servings: 2 glasses

Ingredients:

- 1 cup frozen blueberries
- 1/2 avocado
- 1 cup coconut water
- 1 tablespoon hemp seeds
- 1 tablespoon maple syrup
- Ice cubes (optional)

Directions:

1. Blend frozen blueberries, avocado, coconut water, hemp seeds, and maple syrup until smooth.
2. Add ice cubes for a cooler texture.
3. Pour into glasses and savor the creamy blueberry goodness.

Nutritional Information (per serving):

- Calories: 180
- Protein: 3g
- Fat: 8g
- Carbohydrates: 25g
- Fiber: 7g
- Sugars: 15g

Orange Ginger Carrot Elixir

Prep Time: 12 mins

Total Time: 5 mins

Servings: 2 glasses

Ingredients:

- 3 large carrots, peeled and chopped
- 1 orange, peeled and segmented
- 1/2-inch fresh ginger, peeled and chopped

- 2 cups water
- 1 tablespoon agave nectar or honey
- Ice cubes (optional)

Directions:

1. In a blender, combine chopped carrots, orange segments, fresh ginger, water, and agave nectar.
2. Blend until smooth.
3. Strain if desired and pour into glasses.
4. Add ice cubes for a cooler elixir.

Nutritional Information (per serving):

- Calories: 70
- Protein: 1g
- Fat: 0g
- Carbohydrates: 18g
- Fiber: 4g
- Sugars: 10g

Berry Blast Antioxidant Smoothie

Prep Time: 8 mins

Total Time: 3 mins

Servings: 2 glasses

Ingredients:

- 1 cup mixed berries (blueberries, strawberries, raspberries)
- 1/2 cup ice made with filtered water
- 1 cup almond milk
- 1 tablespoon chia seeds
- 1 tablespoon flaxseeds

- 1 teaspoon honey (optional)
- Handful of fresh mint leaves

Directions:

1. In a blender, combine mixed berries, ice, almond milk, chia seeds, flaxseeds, and honey.
2. Blend until smooth.
3. Garnish with fresh mint leaves.
4. Pour into glasses and enjoy the antioxidant-packed goodness.

Nutritional Information (per serving):

- Calories: 120
- Protein: 4g
- Fat: 6g
- Carbohydrates: 14g
- Fiber: 6g
- Sugars: 6g

Golden Pineapple Turmeric Elixir

Prep Time: 5 mins

Total Time: 2 mins

Servings: 2 glasses

Ingredients:

- 1 cup frozen pineapple chunks
- 1/2 cup ice made with filtered water
- 1 cup coconut water
- 1/2 teaspoon ground turmeric
- 1 tablespoon fresh lime juice
- 1 teaspoon agave nectar

- Pinch of black pepper

Directions:

1. Blend pineapple chunks, ice, coconut water, turmeric, lime juice, agave nectar, and black pepper until smooth.
2. Pour into glasses.
3. Sip on this refreshing elixir and relish the anti-inflammatory benefits.

Nutritional Information (per serving):

- Calories: 90
- Protein: 1g
- Fat: 0.5g
- Carbohydrates: 22g
- Fiber: 2g
- Sugars: 15g

Citrus Ginger Green Tea Cooler

Prep Time: 10 mins

Total Time: 5 mins

Servings: 2 glasses

Ingredients:

- 2 cups brewed green tea, cooled
- 1/2 cup ice made with filtered water
- 1 orange, peeled and segmented
- 1/2-inch fresh ginger, sliced
- 1 tablespoon honey
- Fresh mint leaves for garnish

Directions:

1. In a pitcher, combine brewed green tea, ice, orange segments, ginger, and honey.

2. Stir until honey dissolves.

3. Garnish with fresh mint leaves.

4. Pour into glasses and enjoy the zesty green tea cooler.

Nutritional Information (per serving):

- Calories: 40

- Protein: 1g

- Fat: 0g

- Carbohydrates: 10g

- Fiber: 2g

- Sugars: 8g

Cherry Almond Protein Shake

Prep Time: 5 mins

Total Time: 2 mins

Servings: 2 glasses

Ingredients:

- 1 cup frozen cherries

- 1/2 cup ice made with filtered water

- 1 cup almond milk

- 1 scoop vanilla protein powder

- 1/4 cup almonds

- 1 tablespoon honey (optional)

Directions:

1. Blend frozen cherries, ice, almond milk, vanilla protein powder, almonds, and honey until smooth.

2. Pour into glasses.

3. Indulge in this protein-rich shake that supports joint health.

Nutritional Information (per serving):

- Calories: 180
- Protein: 10g
- Fat: 7g
- Carbohydrates: 23g
- Fiber: 4g
- Sugars: 15g

Pomegranate Berry Bliss Smoothie

Prep Time: 8 mins

Total Time: 3 mins

Servings: 2 glasses

Ingredients:

- 1/2 cup pomegranate seeds
- 1/2 cup ice made with filtered water
- 1 cup mixed berries (blueberries, raspberries)
- 1 cup coconut water
- 1 tablespoon hemp seeds
- 1 tablespoon maple syrup (optional)

Directions:

1. Blend pomegranate seeds, ice, mixed berries, coconut water, hemp seeds, and maple syrup until smooth.

2. Pour into glasses.

3. Savor the delicious blend of antioxidants and nutrients.

Nutritional Information (per serving):

- Calories: 110
- Protein: 3g
- Fat: 3g
- Carbohydrates: 20g
- Fiber: 5g
- Sugars: 12g

SOUP RECIPES

Hearty Vegetable Quinoa Soup

Prep Time: 15 mins

Total Time: 45 mins

Servings: 4 bowls

Ingredients:

- 1 cup quinoa, rinsed
- 1 tablespoon olive oil
- 1 onion, diced
- 2 carrots, sliced
- 2 celery stalks, chopped
- 3 cloves garlic, minced
- 1 can (14 oz.) diced tomatoes
- 6 cups vegetable broth
- 1 teaspoon dried thyme
- 1 teaspoon turmeric powder
- Salt and pepper to taste
- Fresh parsley for garnish

Directions:

1. In a large pot, heat olive oil over medium heat. Add onions, carrots, celery, and garlic. Sauté until vegetables are tender.
2. Add diced tomatoes, vegetable broth, quinoa, thyme, turmeric, salt, and pepper.
3. Bring to a boil, then reduce heat and simmer for 30 minutes or until quinoa is cooked.

4. Garnish with fresh parsley before serving.

Nutritional Information (per serving):

- Calories: 280

- Protein: 8g

- Fat: 5g

- Carbohydrates: 50g

- Fiber: 8g

- Sugars: 6g

Turmeric Ginger Lentil Soup

Prep Time: 10 mins

Total Time: 40 mins

Servings: 4 bowls

Ingredients:

- 1 cup red lentils, rinsed

- 1 tablespoon coconut oil

- 1 onion, finely chopped

- 2 carrots, diced

- 2 teaspoons ground turmeric

- 1 teaspoon ground cumin

- 1 teaspoon fresh ginger, grated

- 6 cups vegetable broth

- 1 can (14 oz) coconut milk

- Salt and pepper to taste

- Fresh cilantro for garnish

Directions:

1. In a large pot, heat coconut oil over medium heat. Add onions, carrots, turmeric, cumin, and ginger. Sauté until onions are translucent.

2. Add red lentils, vegetable broth, and coconut milk. Bring to a boil, then simmer for 30 minutes.

3. Season with salt and pepper. Garnish with fresh cilantro before serving.

Nutritional Information (per serving):

- Calories: 320
- Protein: 13g
- Fat: 15g
- Carbohydrates: 35g
- Fiber: 9g
- Sugars: 4g

Creamy Broccoli Almond Soup

Prep Time: 15 mins

Total Time: 30 mins

Servings: 4 bowls

Ingredients:

- 2 cups broccoli florets
- 1 tablespoon olive oil
- 1 onion, chopped
- 2 cloves garlic, minced
- 1/2 cup almonds, soaked and peeled
- 4 cups vegetable broth
- 1 cup unsweetened almond milk

- Salt and pepper to taste
- Sliced almonds for garnish

Directions:

1. Steam broccoli until tender. Set aside.
2. In a pot, heat olive oil and sauté onions and garlic until golden.
3. Blend almonds with vegetable broth until smooth. Add the almond milk and blend again.
4. Add the almond mixture to the pot, then add steamed broccoli. Season with salt and pepper.
5. Simmer for 15 minutes. Garnish with sliced almonds before serving.

Nutritional Information (per serving):

- Calories: 220
- Protein: 8g
- Fat: 15g
- Carbohydrates: 18g
- Fiber: 6g
- Sugars: 4g

Mushroom Barley Soup

Prep Time: 15 mins

Total Time: 1 hour

Servings: 4 bowls

Ingredients:

- 1 cup pearl barley
- 1 tablespoon olive oil
- 1 onion, diced

- 2 carrots, sliced
- 2 celery stalks, chopped
- 8 oz mushrooms, sliced
- 6 cups vegetable broth
- 1 teaspoon dried thyme
- Salt and pepper to taste
- Fresh parsley for garnish

Directions:

1. Cook barley according to package instructions. Set aside.
2. In a pot, heat olive oil and sauté onions, carrots, celery, and mushrooms until tender.
3. Add vegetable broth, cooked barley, thyme, salt, and pepper.
4. Simmer for 30 minutes. Garnish with fresh parsley before serving.

Nutritional Information (per serving):

- Calories: 280
- Protein: 7g
- Fat: 4g
- Carbohydrates: 56g
- Fiber: 10g
- Sugars: 3g

Tomato Basil Quinoa Soup

Prep Time: 15 mins

Total Time: 45 mins

Servings: 4 bowls

Ingredients:

- 1 cup quinoa, rinsed
- 1 tablespoon olive oil
- 1 onion, chopped
- 2 carrots, diced
- 2 cloves garlic, minced
- 1 can (14 oz) crushed tomatoes
- 6 cups vegetable broth
- 1 teaspoon dried basil
- Salt and pepper to taste
- Fresh basil for garnish

Directions:

1. In a pot, heat olive oil and sauté onions, carrots, and garlic until softened.
2. Add crushed tomatoes, vegetable broth, quinoa, dried basil, salt, and pepper.
3. Bring to a boil, then simmer for 30 minutes or until quinoa is cooked.
4. Garnish with fresh basil before serving.

Nutritional Information (per serving):

- Calories: 250
- Protein: 7g
- Fat: 5g
- Carbohydrates: 45g
- Fiber: 7g
- Sugars: 6g

Anti-Inflammatory Lentil Soup

Prep Time: 15 mins

Total Time: 1 hour

Servings: 4 bowls

Ingredients:

- 1 cup dried green lentils, rinsed
- 1 tablespoon olive oil
- 1 onion, diced
- 2 carrots, sliced
- 2 celery stalks, chopped
- 3 cloves garlic, minced
- 1 teaspoon ground turmeric
- 1 teaspoon ground cumin
- 6 cups vegetable broth
- 1 can (14 oz.) diced tomatoes
- Salt and pepper to taste
- Fresh cilantro for garnish

Directions:

1. In a pot, heat olive oil and sauté onions, carrots, celery, and garlic until softened.
2. Add turmeric, cumin, lentils, vegetable broth, and diced tomatoes.
3. Bring to a boil, then reduce heat and simmer for 45 minutes or until lentils are tender.
4. Season with salt and pepper. Garnish with fresh cilantro before serving.

Nutritional Information (per serving):

- Calories: 320

- Protein: 18g

- Fat: 6g

- Carbohydrates: 55g

- Fiber: 15g

- Sugars: 8g

Ginger Carrot Immunity Soup

Prep Time: 10 mins

Total Time: 30 mins

Servings: 4 bowls

Ingredients:

- 1 lb. carrots, peeled and chopped

- 1 tablespoon coconut oil

- 1 onion, chopped

- 2 cloves garlic, minced

- 1 tablespoon fresh ginger, grated

- 6 cups vegetable broth

- 1 can (14 oz.) coconut milk

- 1 teaspoon ground coriander

- Salt and pepper to taste

- Fresh parsley for garnish

Directions:

1. In a pot, heat coconut oil and sauté onions, garlic, and ginger until fragrant.

2. Add chopped carrots, vegetable broth, coconut milk, and ground coriander.

3. Bring to a boil, then simmer for 20 minutes or until carrots are tender.

4. Season with salt and pepper. Garnish with fresh parsley before serving.

Nutritional Information (per serving):

- Calories: 220
- Protein: 4g
- Fat: 15g
- Carbohydrates: 22g
- Fiber: 6g
- Sugars: 8g

Spinach and Quinoa Superfood Soup

Prep Time: 15 mins

Total Time: 40 mins

Servings: 4 bowls

Ingredients:

- 1 cup quinoa, rinsed
- 1 tablespoon olive oil
- 1 onion, chopped
- 2 carrots, diced
- 3 cups baby spinach
- 6 cups vegetable broth
- 1 teaspoon dried thyme
- 1 lemon, juiced
- Salt and pepper to taste
- Fresh dill for garnish

Directions:

1. In a pot, heat olive oil and sauté onions and carrots until softened.

2. Add quinoa, vegetable broth, thyme, and bring to a boil. Simmer for 20 minutes.

3. Stir in baby spinach and lemon juice. Cook until spinach wilts.

4. Season with salt and pepper. Garnish with fresh dill before serving.

Nutritional Information (per serving):

- Calories: 280
- Protein: 8g
- Fat: 6g
- Carbohydrates: 48g
- Fiber: 7g
- Sugars: 3g

Butternut Squash and Apple Soup

Prep Time: 20 mins

Total Time: 45 mins

Servings: 4 bowls

Ingredients:

- 1 butternut squash, peeled and diced
- 2 apples, peeled and chopped
- 1 tablespoon olive oil
- 1 onion, diced
- 2 teaspoons curry powder
- 6 cups vegetable broth

- 1 can (14 oz) coconut milk
- Salt and pepper to taste
- Toasted pumpkin seeds for garnish

Directions:

1. In a pot, heat olive oil and sauté onions until translucent. Add curry powder and stir.
2. Add butternut squash, apples, vegetable broth, and coconut milk. Simmer for 25 minutes.
3. Blend until smooth. Season with salt and pepper.
4. Garnish with toasted pumpkin seeds before serving.

Nutritional Information (per serving):

- Calories: 290
- Protein: 5g
- Fat: 15g
- Carbohydrates: 38g
- Fiber: 7g
- Sugars: 11g

Miso Mushroom Barley Soup

Prep Time: 15 mins

Total Time: 1 hour

Servings: 4 bowls

Ingredients:

- 1 cup pearl barley
- 1 tablespoon sesame oil
- 1 onion, sliced
- 8 oz. mushrooms, sliced

- 3 tablespoons miso paste
- 6 cups vegetable broth
- 2 green onions, chopped
- Sesame seeds for garnish

Directions:

1. Cook barley according to package instructions. Set aside.
2. In a pot, heat sesame oil and sauté onions until golden. Add mushrooms and cook until tender.
3. Dissolve miso paste in vegetable broth. Add to the pot and bring to a simmer.
4. Stir in cooked barley. Garnish with green onions and sesame seeds before serving.

Nutritional Information (per serving):

- Calories: 260
- Protein: 7g
- Fat: 6g
- Carbohydrates: 48g
- Fiber: 11g
- Sugars: 3g

Turmeric Ginger Carrot Soup

Prep Time: 15 mins

Total Time: 45 mins

Servings: 4 bowls

Ingredients:

- 1 lb. carrots, peeled and chopped
- 1 onion, diced

- 2 cloves garlic, minced
- 1 tablespoon fresh ginger, grated
- 1 teaspoon ground turmeric
- 6 cups vegetable broth
- 2 tablespoons olive oil
- Salt and pepper to taste
- Fresh cilantro for garnish

Directions:

1. In a pot, heat olive oil and sauté onions, garlic, and ginger until fragrant.
2. Add chopped carrots, turmeric, and vegetable broth. Simmer for 30 minutes.
3. Blend until smooth. Season with salt and pepper. Garnish with fresh cilantro before serving.

Nutritional Information (per serving):

- Calories: 160
- Protein: 3g
- Fat: 7g
- Carbohydrates: 22g
- Fiber: 5g
- Sugars: 8g

Quinoa Kale Minestrone Soup

Prep Time: 20 mins

Total Time: 1 hour

Servings: 4 bowls

Ingredients:

- 1 cup quinoa, rinsed
- 1 onion, diced
- 2 carrots, sliced
- 2 celery stalks, chopped
- 3 cloves garlic, minced
- 1 can (14 oz) diced tomatoes
- 6 cups vegetable broth
- 1 cup kale, chopped
- 2 tablespoons olive oil
- Salt and pepper to taste
- Fresh basil for garnish

Directions:

1. In a pot, heat olive oil and sauté onions, carrots, celery, and garlic until softened.
2. Add quinoa, diced tomatoes, and vegetable broth. Simmer for 40 minutes.
3. Stir in chopped kale. Cook until wilted. Season with salt and pepper.
4. Garnish with fresh basil before serving.

Nutritional Information (per serving):

- Calories: 280
- Protein: 9g
- Fat: 7g
- Carbohydrates: 45g
- Fiber: 8g
- Sugars: 5g

Roasted Red Pepper and Lentil Soup

Prep Time: 15 mins

Total Time: 50 mins

Servings: 4 bowls

Ingredients:

- 1 cup red lentils, rinsed
- 2 red bell peppers, roasted and chopped
- 1 onion, diced
- 2 cloves garlic, minced
- 1 teaspoon cumin
- 6 cups vegetable broth
- 2 tablespoons olive oil
- Salt and pepper to taste
- Fresh parsley for garnish

Directions:

1. In a pot, heat olive oil and sauté onions and garlic until translucent.
2. Add red lentils, roasted red peppers, cumin, and vegetable broth. Simmer for 40 minutes.
3. Blend until smooth. Season with salt and pepper. Garnish with fresh parsley before serving.

Nutritional Information (per serving):

- Calories: 220
- Protein: 12g
- Fat: 6g
- Carbohydrates: 30g

- Fiber: 10g
- Sugars: 3g

Mushroom and Barley Soup

Prep Time: 20 mins

Total Time: 1 hour

Servings: 4 bowls

Ingredients:

- 1 cup pearl barley
- 8 oz mushrooms, sliced
- 1 onion, diced
- 3 carrots, diced
- 3 cloves garlic, minced
- 6 cups vegetable broth
- 2 tablespoons soy sauce
- 2 tablespoons olive oil
- Salt and pepper to taste
- Green onions for garnish

Directions:

1. In a pot, heat olive oil and sauté onions, garlic, and mushrooms until tender.
2. Add pearl barley, carrots, soy sauce, and vegetable broth. Simmer for 45 minutes.
3. Season with salt and pepper. Garnish with green onions before serving.

Nutritional Information (per serving):

- Calories: 320

- Protein: 9g
- Fat: 7g
- Carbohydrates: 58g
- Fiber: 13g
- Sugars: 3g

Coconut Spinach Sweet Potato Soup

Prep Time: 20 mins

Total Time: 45 mins

Servings: 4 bowls

Ingredients:

- 2 sweet potatoes, peeled and diced
- 1 can (14 oz.) coconut milk
- 1 onion, diced
- 2 tablespoons red curry paste
- 3 cups baby spinach
- 6 cups vegetable broth
- 2 tablespoons olive oil
- Salt and pepper to taste
- Fresh coriander for garnish

Directions:

1. In a pot, heat olive oil and sauté onions until golden. Add red curry paste and cook for 2 minutes.
2. Add sweet potatoes, coconut milk, and vegetable broth. Simmer for 30 minutes.
3. Stir in baby spinach. Cook until wilted. Season with salt and pepper.

4. Garnish with fresh coriander before serving.

Nutritional Information (per serving):

- Calories: 280

- Protein: 5g

- Fat: 15g

- Carbohydrates: 32g

- Fiber: 6g

- Sugars: 6g

Anti-Inflammatory Lentil Soup

Prep Time: 15 mins

Total Time: 50 mins

Servings: 4 bowls

Ingredients:

- 1 cup dried lentils, rinsed

- 2 carrots, diced

- 2 celery stalks, chopped

- 1 onion, diced

- 3 cloves garlic, minced

- 1 teaspoon ground turmeric

- 6 cups vegetable broth

- 2 tablespoons olive oil

- Salt and pepper to taste

- Fresh parsley for garnish

Directions:

1. In a pot, heat olive oil and sauté onions, garlic, carrots, and celery until softened.

2. Add lentils, turmeric, and vegetable broth. Simmer for 35 minutes.

3. Season with salt and pepper. Garnish with fresh parsley before serving.

Nutritional Information (per serving):

- Calories: 250
- Protein: 15g
- Fat: 7g
- Carbohydrates: 35g
- Fiber: 12g
- Sugars: 4g

Ginger-Turmeric Butternut Squash Soup

Prep Time: 20 mins

Total Time: 40 mins

Servings: 4 bowls

Ingredients:

- 1 medium butternut squash, peeled and diced
- 1 onion, diced
- 2 cloves garlic, minced
- 1 tablespoon fresh ginger, grated
- 1 teaspoon ground turmeric
- 4 cups vegetable broth
- 2 tablespoons coconut oil
- Salt and pepper to taste
- Toasted pumpkin seeds for garnish

Directions:

1. In a pot, heat coconut oil and sauté onions, garlic, and ginger until fragrant.

2. Add butternut squash, turmeric, and vegetable broth. Simmer for 25 minutes.

3. Blend until smooth. Season with salt and pepper. Garnish with toasted pumpkin seeds.

Nutritional Information (per serving):

- Calories: 180
- Protein: 3g
- Fat: 8g
- Carbohydrates: 27g
- Fiber: 5g
- Sugars: 4g

Cauliflower and Broccoli Detox Soup

Prep Time: 15 mins

Total Time: 30 mins

Servings: 4 bowls

Ingredients:

- 1 head cauliflower, chopped
- 1 head broccoli, chopped
- 1 leek, sliced
- 3 cups vegetable broth
- 2 cloves garlic, minced
- 2 tablespoons olive oil
- 1 teaspoon cumin
- Salt and pepper to taste

- Fresh cilantro for garnish

Directions:

1. In a pot, heat olive oil and sauté leeks and garlic until softened.
2. Add cauliflower, broccoli, cumin, and vegetable broth. Simmer for 20 minutes.
3. Blend until smooth. Season with salt and pepper. Garnish with fresh cilantro.

Nutritional Information (per serving):

- Calories: 150
- Protein: 5g
- Fat: 7g
- Carbohydrates: 20g
- Fiber: 8g
- Sugars: 4g

Spicy Tomato Basil Soup

Prep Time: 10 mins

Total Time: 25 mins

Servings: 4 bowls

Ingredients:

- 1 can (28 oz) crushed tomatoes
- 1 onion, diced
- 2 cloves garlic, minced
- 1 teaspoon red pepper flakes
- 4 cups vegetable broth
- 1/4 cup fresh basil, chopped
- 2 tablespoons olive oil

- Salt and pepper to taste
- Grated Parmesan for garnish

Directions:

1. In a pot, heat olive oil and sauté onions and garlic until golden.
2. Add crushed tomatoes, red pepper flakes, and vegetable broth. Simmer for 15 minutes.
3. Stir in fresh basil. Season with salt and pepper. Garnish with grated Parmesan.

Nutritional Information (per serving):

- Calories: 180
- Protein: 4g
- Fat: 9g
- Carbohydrates: 23g
- Fiber: 6g
- Sugars: 12g

Miso Shiitake Mushroom Soup

Prep Time: 15 mins

Total Time: 35 mins

Servings: 4 bowls

Ingredients:

- 1 cup shiitake mushrooms, sliced
- 2 tablespoons miso paste
- 4 cups vegetable broth
- 1 cup baby spinach
- 1 green onion, sliced
- 2 tablespoons soy sauce

- 1 teaspoon sesame oil
- 2 cloves garlic, minced

Directions:

1. In a pot, combine vegetable broth, soy sauce, and miso paste. Bring to a simmer.
2. Add shiitake mushrooms, garlic, and sesame oil. Simmer for 20 minutes.
3. Stir in baby spinach. Cook until wilted. Garnish with sliced green onions.

Nutritional Information (per serving):

- Calories: 120
- Protein: 6g
- Fat: 4g
- Carbohydrates: 16g
- Fiber: 3g
- Sugars: 5g

MEAL PLAN

Day 1

Breakfast: Microbiome Smoothie

Lunch: Ginger-Turmeric Butternut Squash Soup

Dinner: Anti-Inflammatory Lentil Soup

Day 2

Breakfast: Microbiome Smoothie

Lunch: Cauliflower and Broccoli Detox Soup

Dinner: Spicy Tomato Basil Soup

Day 3

Breakfast: Microbiome Smoothie

Lunch: Miso Shiitake Mushroom Soup

Dinner: Ginger-Turmeric Butternut Squash Soup

Day 4

Breakfast: Microbiome Smoothie

Lunch: Spicy Tomato Basil Soup

Dinner: Anti-Inflammatory Lentil Soup

Day 5

Breakfast: Microbiome Smoothie

Lunch: Cauliflower and Broccoli Detox Soup

Dinner: Miso Shiitake Mushroom Soup

Day 6

Breakfast: Microbiome Smoothie

Lunch: Anti-Inflammatory Lentil Soup

Dinner: Ginger-Turmeric Butternut Squash Soup

Day 7

Breakfast: Microbiome Smoothie

Lunch: Spicy Tomato Basil Soup

Dinner: Cauliflower and Broccoli Detox Soup

Day 8

Breakfast: Microbiome Smoothie

Lunch: Miso Shiitake Mushroom Soup

Dinner: Anti-Inflammatory Lentil Soup

Day 9

Breakfast: Microbiome Smoothie

Lunch: Cauliflower and Broccoli Detox Soup

Dinner: Spicy Tomato Basil Soup

Day 10

Breakfast: Microbiome Smoothie

Lunch: Ginger-Turmeric Butternut Squash Soup

Dinner: Miso Shiitake Mushroom Soup

Day 11

Breakfast: Microbiome Smoothie

Lunch: Anti-Inflammatory Lentil Soup

Dinner: Spicy Tomato Basil Soup

Day 12

Breakfast: Microbiome Smoothie

Lunch: Cauliflower and Broccoli Detox Soup

Dinner: Ginger-Turmeric Butternut Squash Soup

Day 13

Breakfast: Microbiome Smoothie

Lunch: Miso Shiitake Mushroom Soup

Dinner: Anti-Inflammatory Lentil Soup

Day 14

Breakfast: Microbiome Smoothie

Lunch: Cauliflower and Broccoli Detox Soup

Dinner: Spicy Tomato Basil Soup

Day 15

Breakfast: Microbiome Smoothie

Lunch: Ginger-Turmeric Butternut Squash Soup

Dinner: Miso Shiitake Mushroom Soup

Day 16

Breakfast: Microbiome Smoothie

Lunch: Anti-Inflammatory Lentil Soup

Dinner: Spicy Tomato Basil Soup

Day 17

Breakfast: Microbiome Smoothie

Lunch: Cauliflower and Broccoli Detox Soup

Dinner: Ginger-Turmeric Butternut Squash Soup

Day 18

Breakfast: Microbiome Smoothie

Lunch: Miso Shiitake Mushroom Soup

Dinner: Anti-Inflammatory Lentil Soup

Day 19

Breakfast: Microbiome Smoothie

Lunch: Cauliflower and Broccoli Detox Soup

Dinner: Spicy Tomato Basil Soup

Day 20

Breakfast: Microbiome Smoothie

Lunch: Ginger-Turmeric Butternut Squash Soup

Dinner: Miso Shiitake Mushroom Soup

Day 21

Breakfast: Microbiome Smoothie

Lunch: Anti-Inflammatory Lentil Soup

Dinner: Spicy Tomato Basil Soup

CONCLUSION

In this comprehensive exploration of an arthritis-friendly lifestyle, we've navigated the seas of understanding, cooking, and savoring meals designed to nurture joint health. From acknowledging the challenges that arthritis presents to delving into the intricacies of nutrition, we've crafted a roadmap for those seeking a balance between health, flavor, and ease of preparation.

Understanding arthritis is crucial to developing a compassionate and informed approach to its management. It's not just a physical ailment but a nuanced experience that intertwines with one's daily life. Our journey began by empathizing with the struggles that individuals face, recognizing that arthritis extends beyond the physical realm into the emotional and psychological domains.

The cornerstone of our approach lies in the recognition that nutrition plays a pivotal role in mitigating arthritis symptoms. Essential nutrients, omega-3 fatty acids, antioxidants, vitamins, and minerals act as the building blocks for joint health. We explored the significance of ingredient substitutions, incorporating healthy fats, low-impact carbohydrates, and lean proteins into daily meals. This information empowers readers to make conscious choices, turning their kitchens into a sanctuary for both pleasure and wellness.

From breakfast to snacks, desserts to beverages, and soups – every meal category was carefully curated to cater to the diverse palate of those with arthritis. These recipes not only prioritize joint health but also celebrate the joy of eating. The emphasis on fresh, whole ingredients provides a refreshing departure from restrictive diets, encouraging a positive relationship with food.

The provided recipes are not just culinary instructions; they are an invitation to partake in a journey of self-care. The Microbiome Smoothie, the centerpiece of our meal plan, symbolizes more than a nutritious drink – it embodies the spirit of embracing holistic well-being. It serves as a reminder that health isn't a destination but a continual process, and every sip contributes to a healthier, happier you. As we conclude this gastronomic exploration, it's essential to acknowledge the resilience and determination of individuals navigating the challenges of arthritis. It's not merely about adapting to a new way of eating; it's a testament to the strength of the human spirit, the ability to find joy in the seemingly ordinary, and the commitment to one's own health.

In the words of Hippocrates, "Let food be thy medicine and medicine be thy food." This ancient wisdom resonates with renewed vigor in our modern understanding of nutrition and its profound impact on health. It's a call to action, an encouragement to view each meal as an opportunity to nourish both body and soul. By making informed and intentional choices, we transform the act of eating into a powerful tool for promoting well-being.

So, dear reader, as you embark on this culinary journey designed for arthritis, remember that you hold the reins of your health. Every ingredient, every recipe, and every meal is a chance to prioritize self-care. May this guide serve as a source of inspiration, guiding you towards a life where joy and health harmoniously coexist.